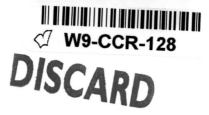

BOMB SQUADS
IN ACTION

Lissette Gonzalez

PowerKiDS press
New York

Published in 2008 by The Rosen Publishing Group, Inc.
29 East 21st Street, New York, NY 10010

Copyright © 2008 by The Rosen Publishing Group, Inc.

First Edition

Editor: Catherine Pearson
Book Design: Greg Tucker
Photo Researcher: Nicole Pristash

Photo Credits: Cover © Tomas del Amo/Index Stock Imagery, Inc.; p. 5 by Dimas Ardian/Getty Images; p. 7 by Koichi Kamoshida/Getty Images; p. 9 by Marty Melville/Getty Images; p. 11 © Ron Brown/Superstock; p. 13 by Dieter Nagl/AFP/Getty Images; p. 15 by Song Kyeong-Seok-Pool/Getty Images; p. 17 by PFC Daniel Klein, USMC; p. 19 by Chip Somodevilla/Getty Images; p. 21 by Aizar Raldes/AFP/Getty Images.

Library of Congress Cataloging-in-Publication Data

Gonzalez, Lissette, 1968–
   Bomb squads in action / Lissette Gonzalez. — 1st ed.
      p. cm. — (Dangerous jobs)
   Includes index.
   ISBN-13: 978-1-4042-3781-0 (lib. bdg.)
   ISBN-10: 1-4042-3781-X (lib. bdg.)
   1. Bomb squads—Juvenile literature. I. Title.
   HV8080.B65G66 2008
   363.17'98—dc22
                                          2006102507

Manufactured in the United States of America

CONTENTS

WHAT ARE BOMB SQUADS?

Bomb squads are teams that are trained to deal with bombs. They take the danger out of **explosives**. Bombs and explosives can hurt people.

People sometimes put bombs, **dynamite**, or other explosives in public places. They make a **threat** to blow up the bombs. This is called a bomb threat. When people hear that there are bombs or explosives around, they get scared. The police usually hear about the scare quickly. That is when a bomb squad gets to do its job.

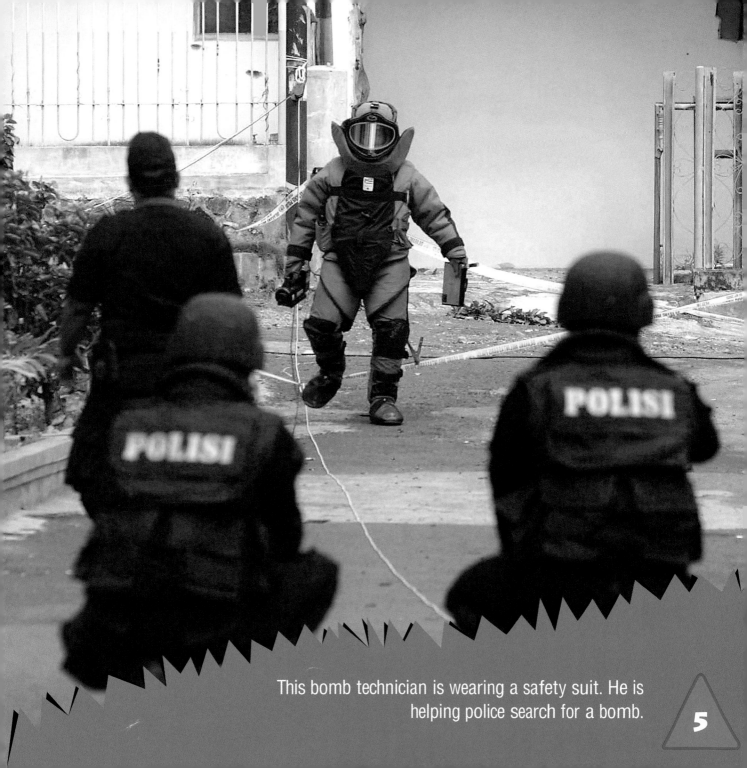

This bomb technician is wearing a safety suit. He is helping police search for a bomb.

SPECIAL TRAINING

People who work in bomb squads are called bomb **technicians**. They know how to take bombs **apart** and keep them from exploding. They know how to use special **equipment** like bomb trucks and machines called bomb robots.

To learn to do their jobs, most bomb technicians go to a special school called the Hazardous Devices School. It has a **mock** village with houses, buildings, streets, sidewalks, parking lots, and even malls! The bomb technicians practice in this village. They treat it like a real town. This way they know just what to do when a real bomb threat happens.

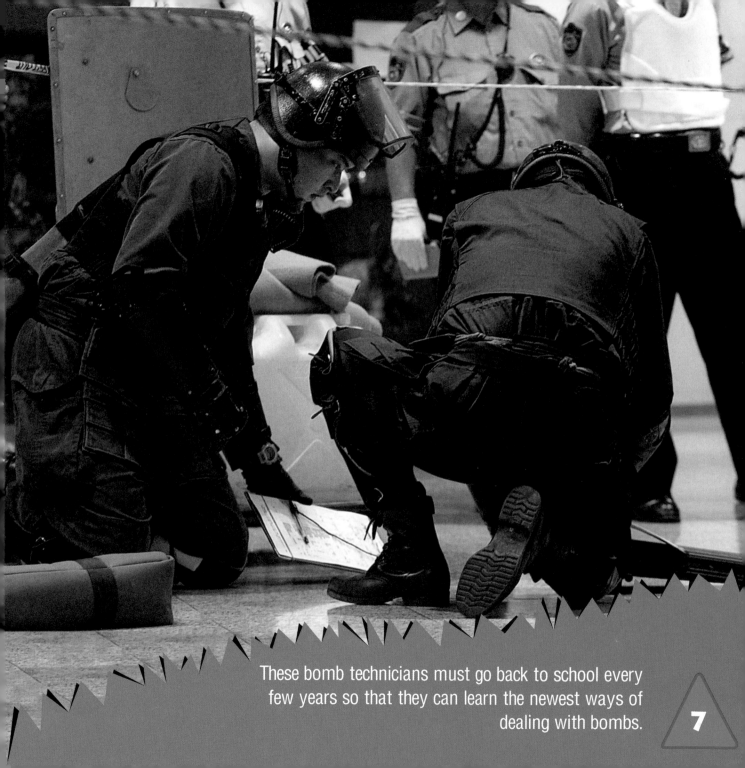

These bomb technicians must go back to school every few years so that they can learn the newest ways of dealing with bombs.

STAYING SAFE

Bomb technicians wear special suits and **helmets** that keep them safe. The suits have plates inside. The plates are made of a hard **material** that stops bomb **debris** from hurting the technicians. Bomb suits can weigh 60 pounds (27 kg) or more. Bomb helmets can weigh almost 15 pounds (7 kg). The helmets have fans inside. The fans cool the technicians so they do not get too hot.

To stay safe on the job, bomb technicians ride in bomb trucks. These are trucks that carry bomb **disposal** equipment. The trucks have special boxes where a bomb can explode without hurting anyone.

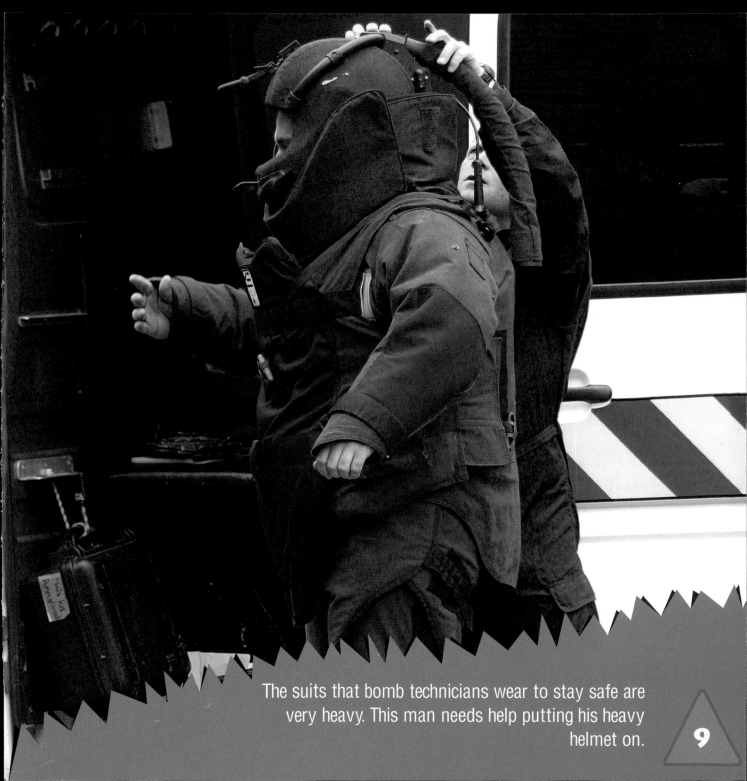

The suits that bomb technicians wear to stay safe are very heavy. This man needs help putting his heavy helmet on.

9

BOMB THREATS

When there is a bomb threat, the first thing that bomb technicians do is search for the bomb. Sometimes there is no bomb. Someone may have made a threat without leaving a bomb. This is called a **hoax**. A hoax threat can be just as scary as a real threat. It is illegal to make a hoax threat, just as it is to make a true threat.

Bomb technicians sometimes use dogs to find bombs. The dogs are trained to find explosives by their smell. Bomb technicians may also use special robots to find bombs. The robots take X-rays to see if something is a bomb. The robots can blow up the bomb without hurting anyone.

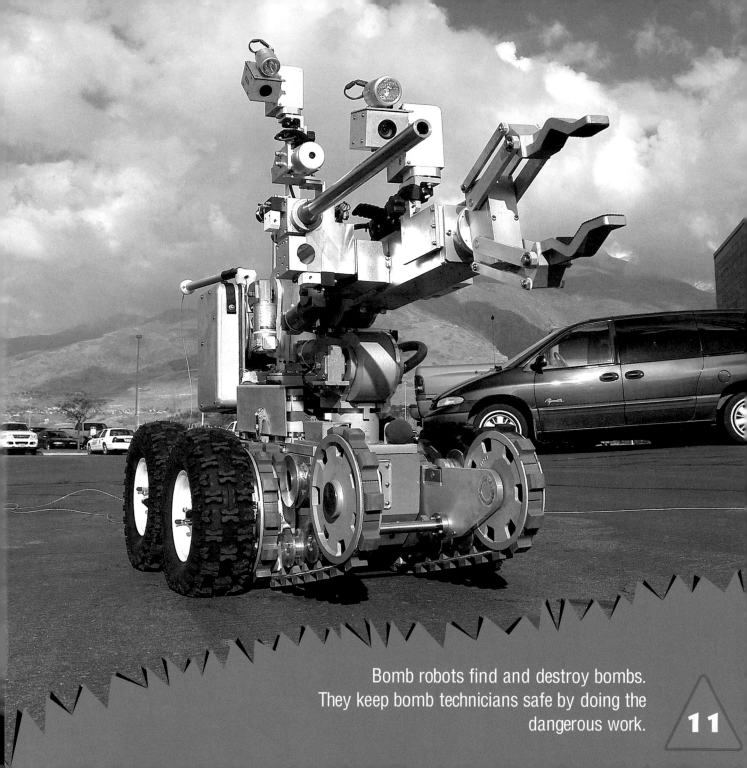

Bomb robots find and destroy bombs. They keep bomb technicians safe by doing the dangerous work.

11

DISMANTLING BOMBS

To dismantle a bomb means to take it apart so that the bomb cannot explode. Sometimes bomb technicians have to dismantle bombs with their own hands. They must do this even if there is a lot of panic and noise around them. They must think only about the bomb.

Bomb squads sometimes blow up bombs remotely instead of dismantling them. "Remotely" means "from far away." The bomb squad first gets everyone away from the bomb. Then the technicians use their own explosives to set off the bomb without hurting anyone.

12

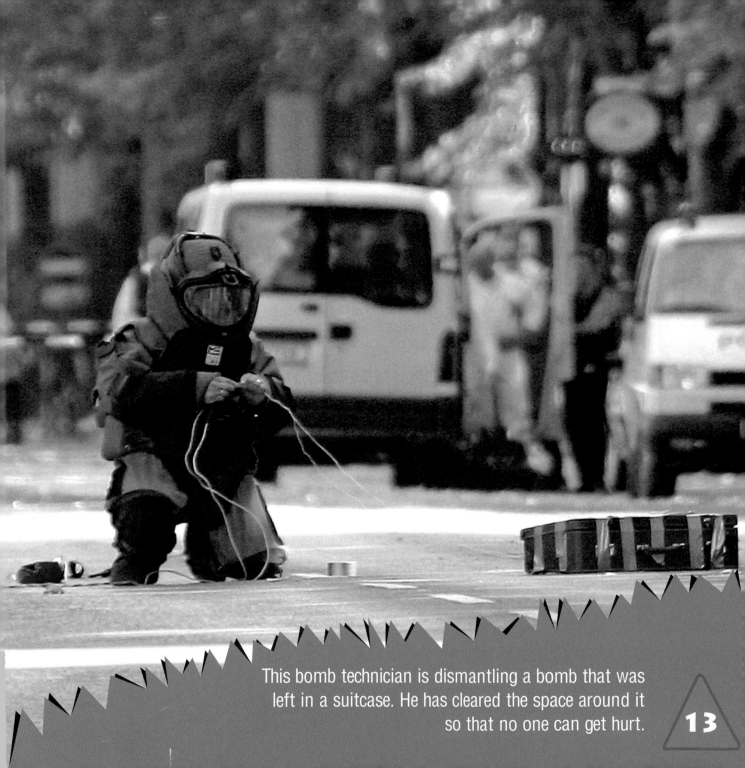

This bomb technician is dismantling a bomb that was left in a suitcase. He has cleared the space around it so that no one can get hurt.

13

HELPING OUT

Bomb squads may be called to help police SWAT teams and police **detectives**. SWAT teams handle problems like **riots**, and they help save hostages. A hostage is a person who is being held by force by someone else. Sometimes bomb threats are made against hostages. SWAT teams can use bomb technicians to dismantle any bombs and free the hostages.

Bomb squads also help **solve** crimes in which explosives are used. Because they know a lot about explosives, bomb technicians can tell police detectives where and how a bomb was made.

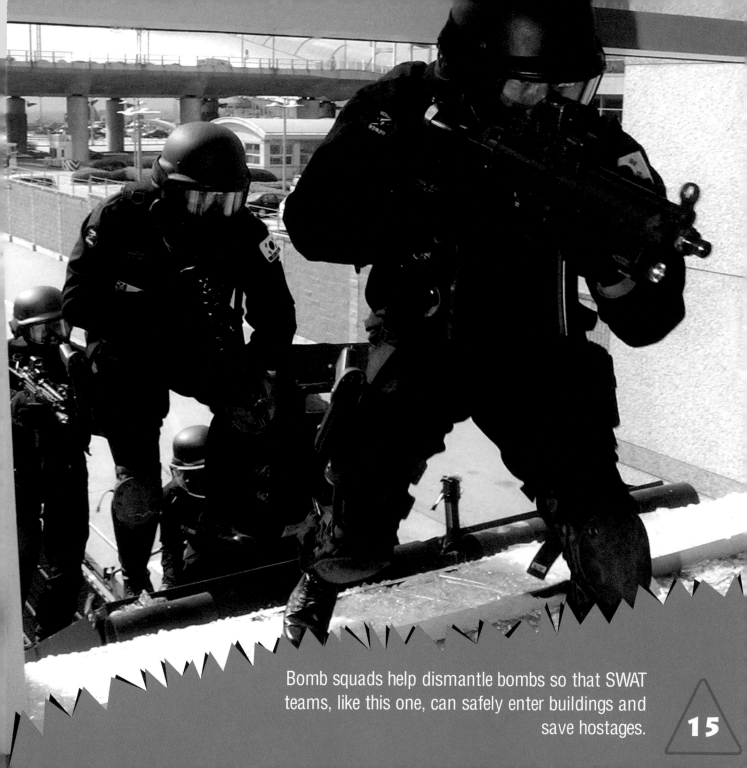

Bomb squads help dismantle bombs so that SWAT
teams, like this one, can safely enter buildings and
save hostages.

15

MILITARY BOMB SQUADS

Military bomb squads are called Explosive Ordnance Disposal troops, or EODs. EODs know how to handle anything from small bombs made at home, to truck bombs, and land mines. Bombs do not always look like bombs. For example, bombs may be put inside soda cans or radios. Military bomb technicians must be ready for anything.

In 2005, a team of three technicians in Iraq called itself Team Mayhem. "Mayhem" means "a lot of disorder." The technicians knew they could handle the mayhem and wanted others to know it, just by hearing the team's name.

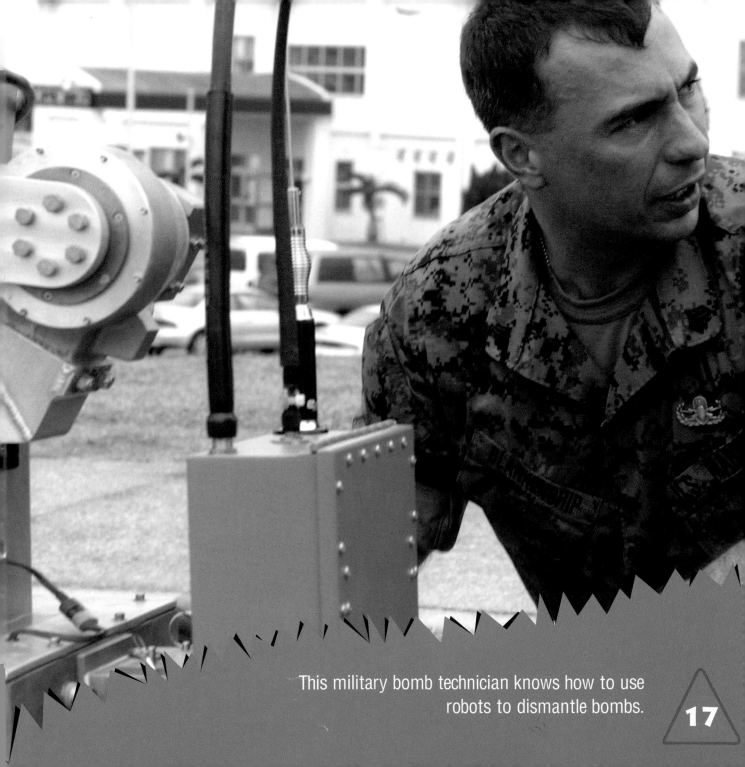

This military bomb technician knows how to use robots to dismantle bombs.

CIVILIAN BOMB SQUADS

Civilians are people who are not in the military. Civilians may work as police officers, firefighters, teachers, or in many other jobs. They can work in bomb squads, too.

Civilian bomb technicians keep people in towns and cities safe. They know that many lives are in danger when a bomb threat is made. In large cities, civilian bomb squads answer many calls every year. The Los Angeles Police Department Bomb Squad answered 1,008 calls in 2005!

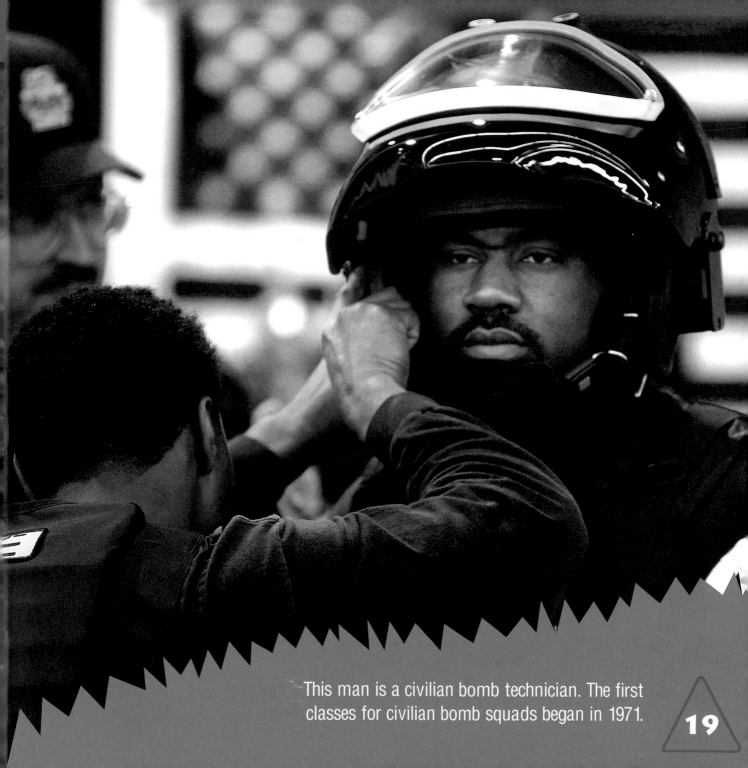

This man is a civilian bomb technician. The first classes for civilian bomb squads began in 1971.

19

DANGEROUS WORK

A bomb explosion can destroy buildings and kill people. Bomb technicians know that they may be hurt while they do their jobs. If they do not dismantle a bomb right away, it may blow up and kill them and many other people.

When bomb technicians are killed on the job, they are remembered with respect. The U.S. military has built the EOD Memorial at Eglin Air Force Base Reserve, in Niceville, Florida. This memorial honors brave military bomb technicians who died while doing their jobs.

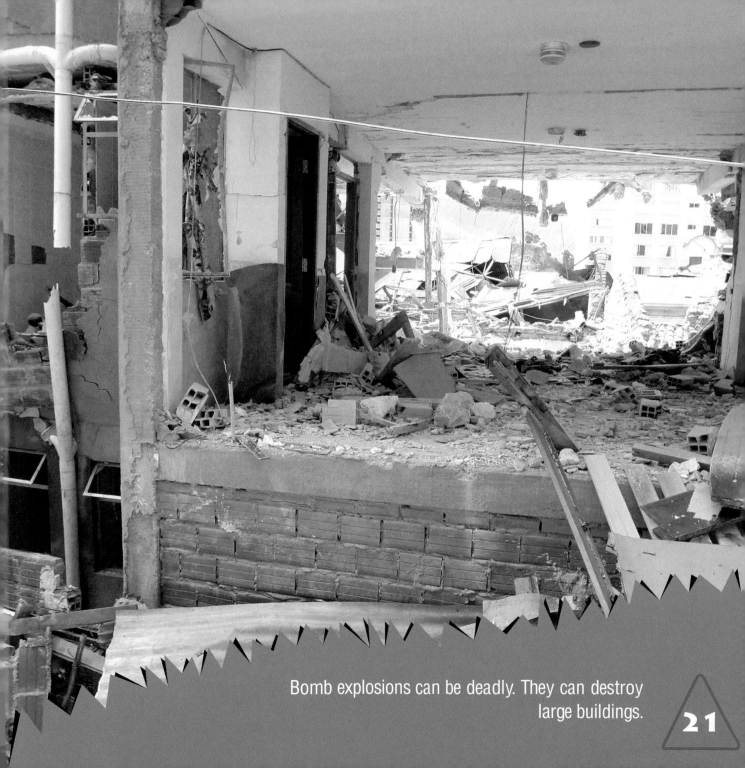

Bomb explosions can be deadly. They can destroy large buildings.

21

WHY BECOME A BOMB TECHNICIAN?

Bomb squads keep people safe in cities and towns all over the country. People trust that bomb technicians will handle bomb threats when they happen. Bomb technicians know that they are trusted and respected in their communities. They like keeping others safe. Bomb technicians also enjoy the **challenges** of their work. They enjoy knowing how to deal with danger. They like knowing how explosives work.

One thing all bomb technicians have in common is their bravery and skill. Bomb squads make it possible for people not to have to live in fear.

22

GLOSSARY

apart (uh-PART) In or into parts or pieces.

challenges (CHA-lenj-ez) Things that require extra effort.

debris (duh-BREE) The remains of something broken down or destroyed.

detectives (dih-TEK-tivz) People who find out the facts and figure out who did a crime.

disposal (dih-SPOH-zul) The act of leaving or getting rid of something.

dynamite (DY-nuh-myt) A powerful explosive used in blasting rock.

equipment (uh-KWIP-mint) All the supplies needed to do something.

explosives (ek-SPLOH-sivz) Things that can blow up.

helmets (HEL-mits) Coverings worn to keep the head safe.

hoax (HOHKS) Something that has been faked.

material (muh-TEER-ee-ul) What something is made of.

mock (MOK) Fake.

riots (RY-uts) Groups of people that are disorderly and out of control.

solve (SOLV) To figure something out.

technicians (tek-NIH-shenz) People who know the special methods of a job.

threat (THRET) A person or thing that may cause others to be hurt or killed.

INDEX

WEB SITES

Due to the changing nature of Internet links, PowerKids Press has developed an online list of Web sites related to the subject of this book. This site is updated regularly. Please use this link to access the list:

www.powerkidslinks.com/djob/bsquad/